Ichraf Ammar
Rania Kalboussi
Nouha Ben Ammar

Mammary tuberculosis

Ichraf Ammar
Rania Kalboussi
Nouha Ben Ammar

Mammary tuberculosis

Literature review

ScienciaScripts

Imprint

Any brand names and product names mentioned in this book are subject to trademark, brand or patent protection and are trademarks or registered trademarks of their respective holders. The use of brand names, product names, common names, trade names, product descriptions etc. even without a particular marking in this work is in no way to be construed to mean that such names may be regarded as unrestricted in respect of trademark and brand protection legislation and could thus be used by anyone.

Cover image: www.ingimage.com

This book is a translation from the original published under ISBN 978-620-6-72540-4.

Publisher:
Sciencia Scripts
is a trademark of
Dodo Books Indian Ocean Ltd. and OmniScriptum S.R.L publishing group

120 High Road, East Finchley, London, N2 9ED, United Kingdom
Str. Armeneasca 28/1, office 1, Chisinau MD-2012, Republic of Moldova, Europe
Printed at: see last page
ISBN: 978-620-8-20583-6

BREAST TUBERCULOSIS: REVIEW OF THE LITERATURE

INTRODUCTION

Mammary tuberculosis is a rare form of extra-pulmonary tuberculosis, even in endemic countries. It accounts for 0.06 to 0.1% of all cases of tuberculosis. The main causative agent, Mycobacterium tuberculosis or Koch's bacillus, is transmitted by air via micro-droplets of mucus called Pflügge droplets expelled by coughing, sneezing and spitting.

This disease can affect many organs, but the lungs are the most common [1].

Mammary tuberculosis ranks last among visceral localisations. It mainly affects women during their childbearing years [2].

However, it must be distinguished from other breast pathologies, especially cancer, given the clinical and radiological similarities. In fact, breast tuberculosis is often mistaken for a cancerous lesion, the diagnosis of which can only be confirmed by anatomopathological and bacteriological examinations [3] .

Treatment is mainly based on anti-tuberculosis drugs, but surgery is sometimes necessary.

RESEARCH STRATEGY

Our searches were carried out in PubMed, google scholar and web of science. We used the following search strategy: (tuberculosis or TB) and (breast). We included studies published in English and French up to the year 2023.

EXTRACTION AND ANALYSIS OF DATA

Each of the included studies was carefully read to extract relevant data. The data extracted included: epidemiological data, general characteristics of the participants, risk factors for breast tuberculosis, type and location of lesions, clinical manifestations, complementary examinations, diagnostic procedures, curative and preventive treatment and prognosis. We emphasise the difficulties involved in making a differential diagnosis with other mastopathies, particularly breast cancer, so as to avoid the need for investigations that can sometimes be mutilating.

A. EPEDEMIOLOGY :

Tuberculosis (TB) is one of the most widespread bacterial infections in the world. In 2018, the WHO reported ten million new cases of TB, the vast majority of them in developing countries [4]. However, mammary tuberculosis (TB mastitis) is not commonly seen in medical practice. It was first described by Sir Astley Cooper in 1829 as a "cold mammary tumour" [5]. The incidence of tuberculous mastitis varies from 0.1% in developed countries to around 4% in highly endemic countries [6,7]. It is generally diagnosed in young multiparous breastfeeding women [8,9].

The term "primary tuberculous mastitis" is used specifically for the rare cases where the tubercle bacillus first infects the breast. Secondary tuberculous mastitis" is used in cases of tuberculosis co-infection elsewhere in the body [10].

Primary mammary tuberculosis is a very rare type of tuberculosis [11]. It occurs in women of childbearing age, but can affect the female breast at any age [14]. Mammary tuberculosis rarely affects men [12]. It accounts for approximately 0.025 to 0.1% of all breast diseases treated surgically [13]. Mammary tuberculosis is more common in developing countries and has a lower incidence in Western countries [11]. Breast tissue is often not a suitable environment for the growth of tubercle bacilli [15].

In Tunisia, mammary tuberculosis is still a very rare form of extrapulmonary tuberculosis, accounting for around 0.2% [17]. Mammary tuberculosis represents 0.025 to 4.5% of all mammary pathologies [18], and its frequency varies according to geographical region.

B. ROUTES OF CONTAMINATION:[19]

Classically, **there are two types** of mammary tuberculosis:

• primary mammary tuberculosis :

This is the form in which the tuberculosis appears to be strictly localised to the breast. It is clearly the most common, accounting for 60% of cases.

However, this opinion is controversial, and some authors believe that other tuberculous foci, mainly scarred pulmonary and intercostal lymph nodes, in fact go undetected, and that this primary form is extremely rare, reserved for cases of direct inoculation.

• secondary mammary tuberculosis :

This is the form in which other organs are affected. This secondary form appears to be much less frequent than the primary form.

There are **five main routes of** tuberculosis **contamination** of the breast:

• the haematogenous route. This route is rarely described. The location of lesions is not determined by the position of vessels, but rather by the structure of the mammary gland. It is lobular and ductal in distribution, as in the lung;

• the lymphatic route. Dissemination of Koch's bacillus occurs retrograde or anterograde from intrathoracic, cervical, supra-clavicular or axillary adenopathies. According to Cooper's theory, communication between the axillary glands and the breast leads to secondary damage to the breast through retrograde lymphatic extension.

• the root canal route. This route of contamination is very rarely observed. The dilatation of the galactophore ducts in women during pregnancy and lactation, as well as locoregional circulatory changes in the course of pregnancy and lactation, are all factors that can lead to contamination. of this period would increase the sensitivity of these ducts to infection, particularly by Koch's bacillus.

• by contiguity. This is the spread of Koch's bacillus from a tuberculous site affecting a rib, the sternum, a cartilaginous site, the sternocostal junction, the lung, the pleura, the chest wall or from an intra-abdominal site.

• the direct route. This is a very rare, if not exceptional, route of contamination. It is the transcutaneous penetration of the bacillus into the breast following a cutaneous or galactophoric abrasion.

C. CLINICAL DIAGNOSIS :

Diagnosis [20] is always difficult because tuberculosis of the breast can mimic a large number of conditions, particularly in elderly women, where breast cancer remains the main concern, but also because of the lack of specificity of its clinical and radiological signs. Only histological evidence can guarantee a definite diagnosis.

However, a few clinical criteria seem useful in drawing attention to a tuberculosis etiology:

• The existence of a breast abscess that recurs after standard antibiotic therapy and correct surgical drainage.

• Fistulised axillary adenopathy associated with a breast nodule.

• Rarely, a mammary fistula with intermittent discharge punctuated by the menstrual cycle.

• Mammary tuberculosis has a variety of clinical features, with an almost always insidious onset that is rarely acute. Lesions are often unilateral, mainly in the quadrant-superolateral region. According to Wilson and MacGregor, only 3% of cases are bilateral (9). Mammary tuberculosis mimics pyogenic abscess in young women and breast carcinoma in older women (10). Three clinical forms are usually described:

• - A nodular form: the most common (75% of patients), it presents as a painless, slowly growing mass in the breast, which may or may not be associated with adenopathy. Mammography reveals a dense lesion with blurred contours, suggestive in the first instance of breast carcinoma (11).

• - A diffuse form with an inflammatory, painful tumour mass, frequently fistulating in the skin. The skin covering is thickened to The lesion and axillary lymph nodes are frequently associated. Mammography initially suggests inflammatory carcinoma (2, 11).

• - A caseous form, more common in older women. This is a painful indurated mass, rarely suppurated (2, 8). Chronic discharge may be observed, but its frequency is assessed differently by different authors. It may be serous, purulent or haemorrhagic. Examination of the lymph nodes reveals axillary lymph nodes in 75% of cases, which are mobile and may progress to fistulisation (12, 13). Cervical adenopathy, homolateral supra-clavicular adenopathy or contralateral axillary adenopathy may also be observed. Adenopathy may precede mammary gland involvement and be the only reason for consultation.

1- Anamnestic data :

a) History:

Risk factors: The risk factors classically reported in the literature are pregnancy, lactation, a history of trauma or breast abscess, chronic mastitis, a history of suppurative breast disease, immunodepression and HIV [21].

History of tuberculosis: The patient's history should include a search for another tuberculosis site, particularly in the lungs, and a history of tuberculosis contagion.

b) Functional signs :

Delays in consultation are frequently observed. In fact, patients
consult after a variable delay ranging from one week to 5 years [18],
which indicates the chronicity of the condition. Mammary
tuberculosis can present in different ways:

Breast swelling: the patient may present with a breast nodule. This is
the most frequent mode of revelation.

Pain: premenstrual mastodynia may be observed.

Breast discharge: a purulent or bloody discharge may be present.
Progression is towards ulceration, with a serous or brownish discharge
with menstrual rhythm.

2- Clinical examination :

Clinically, mammary tuberculosis is characterised by the absence of
specific clinical signs

a) General examination :

Patients are generally in good general condition. This is in the absence
of any other concomitant bacillary localization, particularly in the

lungs, where signs of tuberculosis impregnation are usually found.

b) Breast examination:

** Inspection:

At this stage, morphological changes to the breast are often found. However, the breast may be completely normal. The affected breast as a whole is slightly larger than the opposite breast and has collateral venous circulation. However, its volume may be reduced, particularly in sclerotic forms. The nipple is usually little affected. It may be retracted, but this is a non-specific sign as it is found in all chronic and infiltrating breast lesions. This retraction may appear long before the other signs. There may also be a crusty eczematous ulceration or often multiple ulcerations. The skin opposite the breast is either normal or the site of an inflammatory process giving the appearance of an orange peel. Finally, chronic fistula, which is a rare but more suggestive aspect, may be breast fistula with intermittent discharge or lymph node fistula with a large breast.

** Palpation:

Palpation will show how warm the breast is locally. If there is a lump, its characteristics should be specified:

The shape: is often rounded in cases of tuberculosis [22].

The size: varies from 01 to 10cm [22].

Location: the tumour is frequently located in the upper-external quadrant of the breast. This may be because of the proximity of the axillary lymph nodes. However, other quadrants may also be affected [23-24].

Mammary tuberculosis is often unilateral. Bilateral involvement occurs in 3% of cases [23] .

The boundaries of the mass are usually irregular [23].

Consistency: it can be firm or hard, sometimes stony, simulating breast cancer.

Sensitivity: the tumour is painless in 75% of cases. Occasionally, it is painful and can take on the appearance of a breast abscess or mastitis with a frankly inflammatory appearance.

Mobility: the mass is often mobile and not adherent to the skin or deep layers. It is sometimes adherent, suggesting breast cancer.

Number: tumour masses are often single, multiple nodules are less common.

Palpation will also look for any nipple discharge by concentric pressure of the breast and expression of the nipple. It is necessary to specify the uni or pluriorificial and uni or bilateral character of the discharge, the aspect, the size and the shape of the nipple. quantity and take a sample for a cytological and bacteriological study.

** Examination of lymph nodes:

Palpation of the breasts is followed by palpation of the axillary and supra-clavicular lymph nodes in search of adenopathy, the consistency, size, adhesions, tenderness, location and side affected of which must be specified. According to most authors, lymph nodes are present in 75% of cases. They may be homolateral, contralateral or even bilateral in the axilla, supraclavicular or homolateral in the cervix. They are often unremarkable, mobile and without peri-adenitis. However, they are often larger and more numerous than they would be for a neoplasm of the same size. Over time, these lymph nodes progress towards fistulisation.

D.PARACLINICAL DIAGNOSIS :

1- Radiology :

Mammography in breast tuberculosis is of limited value as the findings are often indistinguishable from carcinoma of the breast [26-27]. The mammographic image of nodular tuberculosis is usually a dense round area with indistinct margins without the classic halo sign found in fibroadenoma [27]. The mammographic size of the tuberculous lesion correlates well with its clinical size, unlike that of a carcinoma [26]. The disseminated variety mimics inflammatory carcinoma and radiographs show a dense breast with thickened skin [27]. Tuberculous sclerosing mastitis appears as a dense homogeneous mass with fibrous septa and nipple retraction [25-26-28-29]. However, as tuberculosis of the breast is common in young women aged between 20 and 40, dense breasts make mammography difficult to interpret.

Ultrasound of the breast is inexpensive and easily accessible, and allows better characterisation of the lesion (particularly cystic lesions) without exposure to radiation [27]. In the nodular form of the disease, lesions are either hypoechoic with poorly defined margins, or complex cystic masses. In diffuse breast tuberculosis, poorly defined hypoechoic masses are seen, whereas in patients with sclerosing breast tuberculosis, increased echogenicity of the breast parenchyma often without a defined mass is seen [27-30]. Occasionally, a beak such as a fistulous connection between the retromammary abscess and the chest wall is seen on ultrasound [36]. Ultrasound examination of the breast enables the effectiveness of medical treatment to be assessed, and also enables ultrasound-guided fine-needle aspiration of deep collections, which avoids the need for multiple punctures [27-28].

Combining mammography and breast ultrasound increases the sensitivity and specificity of both tests.

CT rarely adds to diagnostic yield other than defining chest wall involvement in patients with a deeply adherent breast mass [31]. Tuberculous breast abscess can be considered a hypodense, non-homogeneous lesion with a smooth margin with a surrounding rim on contrast CT. A direct fistulous tract with the pleura or a fragment of rib destroyed in the abscess may also be seen [32]. Percutaneous drainage of a tuberculous breast abscess under CT control is possible [31]. CT may show one or more areas of lung destruction [31-33], and is a valuable tool for demonstrating the extent of the disease.

Breast MRI may reveal a lesion with irregular signal on T2-weighted images suggesting a breast abscess. Again, these findings are not specific and are only useful for demonstrating the extra-breast extent of the lesion [30-32-33].

Chest X-rays are systematic in cases of breast tuberculosis, as active or dormant pleuropulmonary tuberculosis is frequently found [34]. Breast tuberculosis may therefore reveal pleuropulmonary involvement.

A chest X-ray may reveal mediastinal adenopathy, osteitis of the chest wall or pericardial or pleural calcifications. Occasionally, it may show the sequelae of old tuberculosis, often undetected in the form of primary tuberculosis infection, leaving hilar calcifications.

2- Biology: [35]

a. CBC: This may reveal an inflammatory-type anaemia.
Lymphocytosis is found in 40% of cases. Occasionally, the haemogram shows a predominantly neutrophilic hyperleukocytosis.

b.SV: Often accelerated, rarely exceeds 100mm, especially in diffuse inflammatory forms.

b. Tuberculin Intradermal Reaction (TIR): The tuberculin TST or Mantoux test is an interesting test for diagnostic orientation, taking into account the vaccination and immunity profile of the subject.

***Cytology and bacteriology by fine needle aspiration**

- Fine needle aspiration cytology (FNAC) of the breast lesion remains an important diagnostic tool for breast tuberculosis [2].

Approximately 73% of cases of breast tuberculosis can be diagnosed on FNAC by demonstrating the presence of both epithelioid cell granulomas and necrosis [2]. The absence of necrosis on FNAC does not exclude the diagnosis of tuberculosis, given the small quantity o f sample taken and examined.

-Detection of acid-fast bacilli (AFB) on FNAC is not mandatory, as AFB are only seen under the microscope when there are between 10,000 and 100,000 in a millilitre of material [36].

In tuberculous breast abscesses, FNAC may be inconclusive if the specimen is dominated by acute inflammatory exudates. In the case of a BAAR-negative breast abscess which does not heal despite adequate drainage and appropriate antibiotic therapy, the diagnosis of underlying tuberculosis should be made. be suspected. Biopsy of the abscess wall with evidence of the histological characteristics of tuberculosis or a positive culture are essential to confirm the diagnosis of tuberculous mastitis [2-24].

* **Culture** - Although mycobacterial culture remains the gold standard for the diagnosis of tuberculosis, the time required and frequent negative results from paucibacillary samples are major limitations. In addition, culture is not always useful for the diagnosis of mammary tuberculosis [37]. Over the last two decades, several rapid techniques for detecting early mycobacterial growth (5 to 14 days compared with 2 to 8 weeks with conventional methods) have

been described [37], helping to obtain culture and sensitivity reports relatively early. The BACTEC, mycobacterial growth indicator tube (MGIT), Septi-chek and MB / BacT43 systems are among the most important.

*** Polymerase chain reaction (PCR)** - The gene amplification methods (PCR and isothermal) developed for the diagnosis of tuberculosis are highly sensitive, particularly in culture-negative samples from paucibacillary forms of the disease. Various PCR techniques have been developed for the detection of sequences specific to Mycobacleriiiin tuberculosis and other mycobacteria. PCR has positivity rates ranging from 40 to 90% in the diagnosis of tuberculous lymphadenitis [37]. PCR in the diagnosis of mammary tuberculosis is mentioned less frequently, mainly as a tool to distinguish tuberculous mastitis from other forms of granulomatous mastitis in some reports [38]. However, PCR is by no means absolute in the diagnosis of tuberculosis infection and false negatives are always possible [37].

Most of these new techniques are too expensive and sophisticated to be of any practical benefit to the vast majority of TB patients living in underdeveloped countries.

3. Anatomopathological study :

*** Histopathology of the specimen** - Histological findings are consistent with epithcloid cell granulomas with caseous necrosis in the specimen. Basic needle biopsy provides a good sample, often allowing a positive diagnosis. However, open biopsy (incision or excision) of a breast mass, ulcer, or the wall of a cavity suspected of tuberculous breast abscess almost always confirms tuberculosis of the breast [26]. Histologically, tuberculous mastitis is a form of granulomatous inflammation. There are a number of mammary pathologies characterised histologically by a tuberculoid-type tissue reaction. These include sarcoidosis, various fungal infections and granulomatous reactions to modified fats. Sometimes the microscopic picture is indistinguishable from that of tuberculosis [25].

==> Histological classifications [19]

Two classifications are valid for mammary tuberculosis:

Delarue classification: This classification distinguishes four anatomopathological forms:

• Tuberculous mammary lobulitis: this is the most common histological lesion. It affects the glandular lobules, which are the site of caseofollicular lesions with respect for the interlobular canal and perilobular tissues. There are two distinct aspects:

➢ Tuberculous galactophoritis, a lesion that selectively affects the galactophore duct.

➢ Encysted galactophoritis, where the ducts contain thick pus from the calcified wall.

• Vegetative galactophoritis, with intracanal papillary vegetations in the form of fleshy buds containing tubercular follicles;

• cold abscess, which is a suppurated caseous focus, open or not in a galactophore and containing pus with BK ;

• miliaria of the breast. This is an exceptional location for generalised granulosis, characterised by several isolated, pinhead-sized, yellowish-white foci. Histologically, the intralobular lesion has all the features of tubercular miliaria.

McKeown and Wilkinson classification: The most widely used, mammary tuberculosis is divided into five different types, nodular tuberculous mastitis, disseminated tuberculous mastitis, sclerosing tuberculous mastitis, obliterative tuberculous mastitis and acute military tuberculous mastitis. The nodulocaseous form presents as a painless, slow-growing, well-circumscribed mass that progresses to involve the overlying skin and may ulcerate, forming discharged sinuses. The disseminated form begins with multiple foci throughout the breast, causing sinus formation with or without painful ulceration. The sclerosing form occurs in the elderly, the dominant feature being excessive fibrosis rather than caseation. Tuberculous mastitis obliterans is characterised by infection of the ducts causing proliferation of the mucosal epithelium with marked epithelial and periductal fibrosis. Acute miliary tuberculous mastitis is considered to be part of generalised miliary tuberculosis [39].

E. Differential diagnoses: [18,40]

1. Breast cancer :

Breast cancer poses the greatest differential diagnostic problem with mammary tuberculosis. Tuberculous mastitis, especially in its nodular form, gives rise to fears of cancer. In the case of mammary carcinoma, nipple retraction and discharge are more frequent than in the case of tuberculosis.

Axillary adenopathy in cases of mammary tuberculosis is usually unremarkable. However, they are larger and more numerous than they would usually be for a neoplasm of the same volume.

Inflammatory breast cancer can be confused with acute breast tuberculosis, as can pyogenic breast suppurations. Clinically, it is possible to orientate more towards the benign nature of tuberculosis, by grouping together a certain number of criteria as follows:

• The terrain, with multiparity, pregnancy, breastfeeding and the patient's young age;

• Purulent galactorrhoea ;

• Localised pain ;

• Mammary fistulas ;

• An extra-mammary tuberculosis site;

• An intact nipple;

However, certainty is based on the demonstration of epithelioid and giganto-cellular granulomas on pathological examination.

2. Mammary abscess: This is the main problem of differential diagnosis in young women. The diagnostic approach varies in difficulty depending on whether the mastitis is acute or chronic.

-Acute mastitis: the clinical appearance, especially at the beginning of the course, is very similar to that of an acute breast abscess and mammary tuberculosis. Cytopuncture is the key to diagnosis and shows the lesion to be pyogenic, with a staphylococcal culture.

-Chronic breast abscess: This is a major problem when differentiating infectious mastitis from tuberculosis. A bacteriological study of the pus must be carried out in order to eliminate a germ. In addition, whenever the pus is amicrobial, a search for tuberculosis should be carried out systematically, particularly in endemic countries.

3. Benign mastopathies :

a. Fibroadenoma: this is a common breast tumour in young women. It is a solid, elastic, well circumscribed and mobile lesion, which can appear in any part of the breast and is generally multiple and tends to recur after removal.

b. Fibrocystic disease: covers a wide range from cysts with an epithelial border to sclerosing adenomas, presenting as a well-circumscribed, fluctuating mass. In the case of a solid tumour, the tenderness of the mass may suggest a solid tumour, but conversely, its softness and the notion of a sudden appearance are in favour of a cyst. A patient presenting with small diffuse cystic abnormalities, with a significant fibrous reaction and nodular, painful breasts, poses a problem of differential diagnosis with mammary tuberculosis.

4. Granulomatous mastitis: This is a benign and rare condition, accounting for 0.5% of breast tumours. It is a chronic inflammatory lesion, amicrobial, localised to the lobules and affecting the proximal subareolar galactohoric ducts, which affects young women. Histological examination confirms the diagnosis, showing diffuse inflammatory lesions and nodular formations: the "granuloma", composed of Langerhans-type giant cells or "foreign body reaction" cells and epithelioid cells without caseous necrosis. The granuloma is extra-areolar.

5. Plasma cell mastitis: Plasma cell mastitis is a benign, antimicrobial disease of the breast characterised by plasma cell infiltration. It affects 25 to 40% of women over the age of 50.

F. Treatment:

There are no specific guidelines for treating breast tuberculosis. The disease is treated like any other form of extrapulmonary tuberculosis. Usually, anti-tuberculosis treatment is the primary treatment for breast tuberculosis and minimal surgery is performed to remove residual lesions. Anti-tuberculosis treatment includes rifampicin, isoniazid, pyrazinamide and ethambutol [5]. Recovery is usual, although often delayed. Mastectomy is reserved for patients with persistent residual infection [18].

G. Evolution :

a- No treatment:

The most common course is suppuration. Progression is either slow or accelerated by pregnancy or breast-feeding. The mastitis becomes softer and fluctuates. If the mass is left alone, an intramammary cold abscess builds up and eventually adheres to the superficial surface, causing skin and nipple retraction and then fistulation to the skin, leaving in place, after partial evacuation, a characteristic chronic tubercular fistula with a single or, more frequently, multiple openings. Finally, the breast becomes irregular, bumpy and fistulated at several points.

b- Under treatment:

The outcome is favourable when treatment is early and well-administered.

c- Surveillance:

-Clinical: including general examination, weight, breast examination and examination of all lymph nodes. It also includes a pleuropulmonary examination and assessment of tolerance to anti-tuberculosis drugs.

-Organic: by VS

Radiological: mammography, breast ultrasound and chest X-ray.

E. Prognosis:

The patient's life is not compromised when mammary tuberculosis is isolated. In other words, the patient's vital prognosis depends on other tuberculosis sites, which must be systematically investigated with the utmost care.

F. Prevention :

1. Contact prevention measures: isolation of the contaminated patient;

2. Vaccination;

3. Chemoprophylaxis: Isoniazid-based chemoprophylaxis for 6 to 9 months at a dose of 5 mg/kg/day, not to exceed 300mg/day:

• Subjects with latent tuberculosis infection.

• HIV+ subjects

• Newborn infants if the mother is contagious at birth and if there are

no clinical or radiological signs of active tuberculosis.

CONCLUSION

Mammary tuberculosis is a rare extra-pulmonary site of tuberculosis, the diagnosis of which can pose a number of clinical and paraclinical difficulties. It is only confirmed by histological study of the biopsies, which show lesions specific to tuberculosis: the presence of "epithcloid cell granulomas with caseous necrosis". The essential differential diagnosis is breast cancer, which should never be overlooked. Despite its rarity, this diagnosis should be considered in countries where tuberculosis is highly endemic, such as Tunisia.

REFERENCES

[1] Updates in tuberculosisAuthor links open overlay panelAnaïsDupont(Pharmacien d'officine)aChetaouMahaza(Professeur des universités)bVéroniqueApaire-Marchais(Professeur des Universities, attached practitioner)

[2] Agoda-Koussela. L.K, Djibril. A .M, Adjessou. K.V ; Tuberculosis of the breast: A case report. J Afr Imag Méd 2014; 6 (3),73-77... [3]

Zekri.H, Boufettal.H,Bennairi .Oen collaboration ; La tuberculose mammaire à propos de dix cas .Journal Marocain des Sciences Médicales 2010, Tome XVII ; N°2, 19-22.

[4] Global Tuberculosis Report 2019

World Health Organization (Ed.) , World Health Organization (2019)

[5] Illustrations of Breast Diseases Longman, California, & Rees, O. Brown and Green , London (1829)

[6] .R. De Sousa , R. Patil Mammary tuberculosis or granulomatous mastitis: a diagnostic dilemma Ann. Trop. Med. Santé publique , 4 (2) (2011) , p. 122

[7] .S. Gon Tuberculous mastitis - A great masquerade / Tüberküloz

Mastiti- Büyük Taklitçi Turkish. J. Pathol. , 29 (1) (2013) , pp. 61 - 63

[8].PT Kao , MY Tu , SH Tang , HK Ma Tuberculosis of the breast with erythema nodosum: a case report J. Med. Case Rep. , 4 (1) (2010) , p. 124

[9].SR Shinde , RY Chandawarkar , SP Deshmukh Tuberculosis of the breast disguised as carcinoma: a study of 100 patients World J. Surg. 19 (3) (1995) , pp. 379 - 381

[10].G. Schaefer Tuberculosis of the breast: a review with the additional presentation of ten cases Un m. Rev. Tuberc. Pulmonary Dis. 72 (6) (1955) , pp. 810 - 824

[11].G. Madhusudhan Ks Primary breast tuberculosis disguised as carcinoma Singapore Med. J. , 49 (1) (2008)

[12].C. Jaideep , M. Kumar , AK Khanna Male mammary tuberculosis Postgrad. Med. J. 73 (861) (1997) , pp. 428 - 429

[13].N. Kalarç , B. Ozkan , H. Bayiz , AB Dursun , F. Demirağ Breast Tuberculosis Breast , 11 (4) (2002) , pp. 346 - 349

[14].PP Rosen Specific Infections Rosen's Breast Pathology (4th ed.) , Lippincott Williams and Wilkins (2015)

[15].SP Luh , JD Hsu , YS Lai , SW Chen Primary tuberculous breast

infection: experiences of surgical resection in elderly patients and review of t h e literature J. Zhejiang Univ. Sci. B , 8 (8) (2007) , pp. 580 - 583

[16].PP Gupta , KB Gupta , RK Yadav , D. Agarwal Tuberculous mastitis: review of seven consecutive cases Indian J. Tuberc. 50 (1) (2003) , pp. 47 - 50

[17] Direction des soins de santé de base. Ministry of Public Health. Republic of Tunisia. Bull Epidemiol 2001;23:9-10.

[18] Khaiz D, Lakhloufi A, Chehab F, et al. Mammary tuberculosis. About two cases. Sem Hop Paris 1993;69:454-8

[19] . Mammary tuberculosis: a retrospective study of 65 cases Author links open overlay panelJ.BenHassounaaA.GamoudibH.BouzaieneaT.DhiabaF.KhomsiaR. Chargui a

H.SifiaM.MtaallahaR.MakhloufaA.ChebbicH.BoussendM.Héchichea K.Rahala

[20] Ben Hassouna . J et Al ; Gynécologie obstétrique et fertilité 33, (2005) ,870876.

[21]. J.J.C. Rajaonarison, J.M. Rakotondraisoa, B.S. Rasoanandrianina, E. Ravelosoa, D.M.A. Randriambololona. A new

case of primary mammary tuberculosis. Rev. méd. Madag. 2015; 5(1): 534-537).

[22] Mahjoub H. Mammary tuberculosis. Thesis for Doctorate in Medicine Tunis 1992: n° 111.

[23] WILSON J.P., CHAPMAN S.W.Tuberculous mastitis, Chest 1990; 98:1505 1509.

[24] EI MANSOURI A., MOUMEN M., LOUAHLIA S. Tuberculosis mammary: three cases, Sem. Hop. Paris 1993;69:12771279. [25]. Banerjee SN, Ananthakrishnan N, Mehta RD, Prakash S. Tuberculous mammitis: a persistent problem. World J Surg 1987; 11: 105-9. [26]. Shinde SR, Chandawarkar RY, Deshmukh SP. Tuberculosis of the breast masquerading as carcinoma: a study of 100 patients. World J Surg 1995; 19: 37981.

[27]. Popli MB. Pictorial essay: tuberculosis of the breast. Indian J Radiol Imag 1999; 9: 127-32.

[28]. Schnarkowski P, Schmidt D. Kessler M, Reiser MF. Tuberculosis of the breast: US, mammographic and CT findings. J Comput Assist Tomogr 1994; 18: 970- 1.

[29]. Makanjuola D. Murshid K, Al Sulaimani S, Al Saleh M. Mammographic features of mammary tuberculosis: skin bulge and sinus tract sign. Clin Radiol 1996; 51: 354-8.

[30]. Oh KK, Kim JH, Kook SH. Imaging of tuberculous disease of the breast. Eur Radiol 1998; 8: 1475-80.

[31]. Romero C, Carreira C, Cereceda C, Pinto J, Lopez R, Bolanos F;. Mammary tuberculosis: percutaneous treatment of a mammary tuberculous abscess. Eur Radiol 2000; 10: 531-3.

[32]. Bhatt GM, Austin HM. The CT demonstration of empyema necessitates. J Coinput Assist Tomogr 1985; 9: 1108-09.

[33]. Chung SY, Yang I, Bae SH, Lee Y, Park HJ, Kim HH, et al. Tuberculous abscesses in the rctromammary region: CT findings. J Comput Assist Tomogr 1996; 20: 766-9.

[34]) AINAB I, IDRISSI A, ZAMIATI W, ADIL A. Radiological aspects of mammary tuberculosis

[35] SOPENA B.,MIRAMONTES S., CLIMENT A., GARCIA-VILA LM ARNILLAS Tuberculosis of the breast: unusual clinical presentation of extrapulmonary tuberculosis

[36]. Pagel W, Simmonds FAH, Macdonald J, Nassau E. Pulmonary Tuberculosis. 4th ed. London: Oxford University Press; 1964 p. 245.

[37]. Katoch VM. New diagnostic techniques for tuberculosis. Indian J Med Res 2004; 120: 418-28.

[38]. Tse GM, Poo \ n CS, Ramachandram K, Ma TK, Pang LM, Law

BK, et al. Granulomatous mastitis: a clinicopathological review of 26 cases. Pathology 2004; 36: 254-7.

[39].KC Mckeown , KW Wilkinson Tuberculous breast disease Br. J. Surg. 39 (157) (1952) , pp. 420 - 429

[HERRMAN JL, LAGRANGE P. Bacteriology of tuberculosis and atypical mycobacterial infections. EMC, Pneumology 1999; 6-019-A34.

SUMMARY

Mammary tuberculosis: review of the literature

Introduction

Mammary tuberculosis is a rare form of extrapulmonary tuberculosis, even in endemic regions, accounting for only 0.06% to 0.1% of all tuberculosis cases. Caused by Mycobacterium tuberculosis, it mainly affects the lungs, but can spread to other organs, including the breast. Mammary tuberculosis, which is often confused with a malignant tumour due to its clinical and radiological similarities, mainly affects women of childbearing age. Diagnosis is based on bacteriological and histopathological evidence, and treatment is mainly based on anti-tuberculosis drugs, with surgery sometimes necessary.

Methods

A literature review was carried out using the PubMed, Google Scholar and Web of Science databases. The search terms used were "tuberculosis" and "breast", and studies published up to 2023 in English and French were included. Data retrieved covered epidemiology, clinical features, risk factors, diagnostic difficulties, therapeutic approaches and prognosis. Particular attention was paid to the difficulties of differentiating between breast tuberculosis and other breast pathologies, particularly cancer, in order to avoid unnecessary invasive procedures.

Results

Mammary tuberculosis is a rare occurrence, accounting for 0.025% to 4.5% of all cases. of all breast pathologies in Tunisia. The majority of patients are young, multiparous women. The disease presents in primary or secondary forms, with the primary form being extremely rare. The Clinical manifestations include breast masses, pain or purulent discharge. Imaging examinations, such as mammography and ultrasound, often mimic malignant pathology, but the diagnosis is confirmed by cytological or histopathological examination, revealing granulomatous inflammation with caseous necrosis. Fine needle aspiration (FNAC) and biopsy are essential for an accurate diagnosis.

Discussion

Mammary tuberculosis poses a major diagnostic challenge due to its non-specific clinical presentation and radiological overlap with breast cancer. The main risk factors include pregnancy, breastfeeding, immunosuppression and a history of exposure to tuberculosis. Differential diagnosis includes breast cancer, abscesses, fibroadenomas and granulomatous mastitis. Treatment is mainly based on multi-drug antituberculosis therapy (isoniazid, rifampicin, pyrazinamide and ethambutol) for six months. Surgery is reserved for complex cases, such as abscesses, or when treatment fails. The prognosis is generally favourable if treatment is started early.

Conclusion

Although rare, breast tuberculosis should be considered in the differential diagnosis of breast lesions, particularly in endemic regions. Early diagnosis and appropriate treatment can prevent complications. The main diagnostic challenge lies in distinguishing between tuberculosis and breast cancer, but histopathological confirmation remains the gold standard for diagnosis. Appropriate treatment generally leads to a complete cure, underlining the importance of early treatment.

Key words: breast; tuberculosis; mammography; ultrasound; disease;

treatment.

TABLE OF CONTENTS

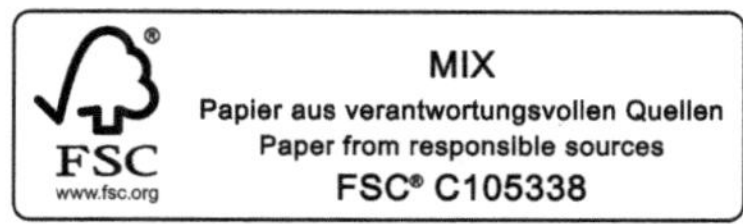

Printed by Books on Demand GmbH, Norderstedt / Germany